60 Holistic ways to get slim and stay slim

Never diet again

By Katrina Zawawi
Kundalini with Katrina

About the Author

I'm Katrina Zawawi. I run Kundalini with Katrina, which is all about helping people overcome trauma and stress by being in charge of their health. Kundalini with Katrina is all about focusing on good nutrition and yogic teachings. The aim is to be able to manage stress and be healthy, physically, emotionally and mentally.

I suffered stress most of my life. I felt inadequate growing up and was overweight as consequence of that. I also suffered intense eczema, asthma and sinusitis. Now, thanks to my change in lifestyle, my health is all good, apart from the odd eczema flare up (usually caused by environmental allergens).

I have been on many diets,Weight Watchers, Atkins, The 5:2 diet, and many more. Some were crash diets, and others were low calorie meals. After the novelty of dieting wore off, all of these diets involved a great amount of control and willpower. Like a tight rubber band ready to ping, I pinged as soon as I reached a frustrating plateau. You can guess what happened - yes! I gained all the weight back, and more. Diet after diet, regime after regime, it was all about control. My life seemed to be about not eating this, not eating that, avoiding parties and avoiding social events in general. It was painful. But what was worse was that in between the diets, my eczema flared, as did my asthma, and I was feeling rotten inside. So, that was really not a way to live. I needed to find another way.

After my divorce, I felt that I could live my life the way I wanted to, so I began to research, study and learn what I could about nutrition. My partner, Ed, who is now our in-house nutritionist in Kundalini with Katrina, was on his own personal journey to correct his diet too. I took up several online courses in health, fitness and nutrition, whilst practicing Bikram yoga. I found the Bikram yoga detoxed me from alcohol and sugary foods, and gave me the desire to go plant based.

It was through years of hard work, losing some weight, then gaining it again, changing my diet a little bit here and there that I learned what worked and what didn't for my health and wellbeing. On my own journey, I learned to let go of the weight loss as a goal, focus on health and on the deepest desire behind the weight loss.

When I peeled it back, I discovered that the fear of diabetes was the driving force. So, that was when I decided to embark on my health journey. I was going to make sure that whatever I do, I will keep diabetes at bay. Since deciding that, I have maintained the size that I am.

I learned by focusing on healthy nutrition, managing my stress levels and my asthma, sinusitis and eczema pretty much vanished. The most welcomed side effect to that was weight loss.

Your slimming journey is personal to you. This book will give you some very useful tools that mean you never have to feel compelled to diet or do intense exercise to achieve health. And yes, the weight/fat loss is a very welcome side effect.

Before you begin, you must let go of weight being your goal. If you don't, it will cause you to feel more stress in your mind. If you make a specific health is-

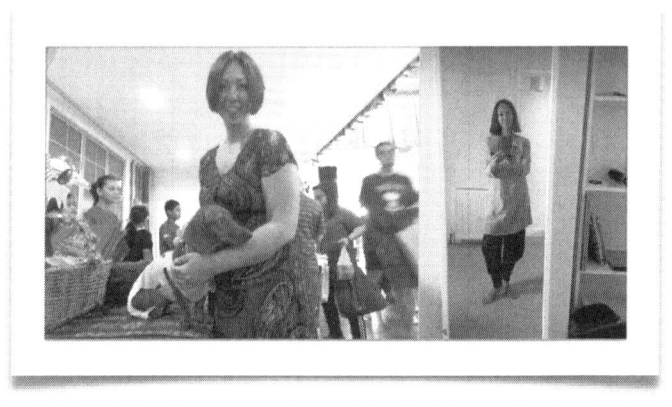

Above left was me before I embarked on a journey that used stress management and nutrition as a tool for health. On the right, you can see my size reduction. On my journey, I never weighed myself nor controlled my eating. I ate when I was hungry and exercised regularly. That was it. My change in mindset was the only difference compared to all of the other times that I tried dieting before. This time it was effortless, and I still don't know what my weight is. But I'm how I want to look and I am happy and healthy.

sue a priority, fat loss will be a positive outcome. What is your health priority?

Acknowledgements

I would like to say thank you to the members of the Facebook groups, 'Breaking Patterns of Narcissistic Abuse through finding Relief to Love' and 'Kundalini with Katrina'. You have all motivated me one way or another to share my knowledge and experiences around approaching fat loss from the perspective of stress management. I would love to thank all my clients for their inspiration and hard work. Much of what I have learned has been through trial and error - the journey that I share in this book. My clients taught me how different we all are and how each person's individuality has to matter when trying to lose fat. I won't mention names, but there is a particular client I would like to thank for making me aware of how dangerous it is to monitor weight. I have learned that the issues constant weight-watching brings are highly connected to mental health as well - which is also very much linked to obsession and obsessive compulsive disorder (OCD).

I would love to also say a big thank you to Jonny Cooper, of 'Jonny hates Marketing' fame. Having read his book on marketing as well as receiving his daily emails on brain tattoos I was inspired. It made me realise: why not combine everything I know and understand and have learned on my journey with my clients into a book? Thank you Jonny, for that.

I want to share my gratitude to my yogic teachers and friends for teaching me how to love myself and how to let go of the irrelevant stuff. I learned so much during the Indian lockdown experience about letting go of stuff. Surrendering to the universe has been a big part of how I live now, and it has prevented me from getting stressed like I used to and has kept my weight in balance. Thank you for teaching me and for your continuous support and guidance.

I am also grateful to my friends and family for their belief in me and keeping me motivated to pursue any dreams I have, without judgement. Johann, you have taught me so much through your challenges as someone on the Autism spectrum. I really make mental health a priority in everything that I do, because you have taught me how important it is. To Aslan and his beautiful family, you have taught me how to listen more than speak. You are very calm, even though you are the youngest of all three of us, and the most patient.

I would love to show gratitude to my Mum and Dad for their ongoing love and support through my journey through life, and particularly to India recently, not to mention supporting myself and my partner through our darkest moments there. I know my mum wasn't entirely happy about me going out to India but she still backed me up, because it was something I wanted and needed to do, and she respected that. You have continued to support me more than you know. I love you both so much.

Finally, I am extremely thankful and blessed to be with Edward, my partner who has stuck by me the whole time since 2017. Ed is the plant-based nutritionist in Kundalini with Katrina and we are partners in business, in our jazz duo and soul partners too. We were both stuck on lockdown in a tiny bedroom in Rishikesh, India for several months. That didn't kill our relationship but taught us to show more respect and gratitude for one another. Ed has seen me at my best and worst, and accepts all of me in the way I truly am. I am authentic with him. Edward, you are my rock, and I wouldn't want to samba through life without you. I love you.

Chapter 1: Get inquisitive - Become your own scientist

Find out what you are about. We are all different, what works for some doesn't work for others.

- Start journaling your emotions and your foods

- According to Dr. Jade Teta, integrative physician, you need to focus on how much sleep are you getting. Is it 8 hours or more? How hungry are you throughout the day? Do you eat until you feel satiated, but not full? What is your mood like through the day? Do you feel emotional, angry, frustrated? How much energy do you have throughout the day? What foods do you crave? All of this should be in balance to ensure your hormones are in balance, so you can lose fat easily.

- Find out what works through the **process of elimination; eliminate** the foods that you may be allergic to, find out what gives you an inflammatory response or makes you feel unwell afterwards.

- For instance, could you have unknown food allergies? Many people are allergic to dairy and gluten. This is worth looking into.

- Go for an allergy test.

- After eating, do you feel sleepy? If you do, you are eating foods that are harder to digest, and the body needs to use all its energy to do this. Make a note of this.

- Make note of how you feel after binge-eating, binge-drinking or indeed anything else excessive that most people regard as fun! Just because it is widely accepted does not mean it will agree with your body.
- How do processed foods make you feel?

Be inquisitive about each change of eating habit and lifestyle.

Always ask yourself, How does ………. make me feel? You are you, not anyone else.

Chapter 2: Cut out Ultra-processed foods/Junk foods - Or at least limit them

Junk Foods and Ultra Processed Foods are addictive. Try to cut them out of your lifestyle. Or at least, limit them to (rare) special occasions.

- Did you know that these foods have been scientifically processed to look good, and carefully adapted to create the perfect taste, crispness, softness, creamyness?

- Did you know that all Ultra processed/Junk foods **increase hormones in your body that prevent you from feeling full**, even though you already are?

- They therefore **increase the appetite for more of these foods.**

- Have you ever salivated over raw broccoli? Have you ever been dying for an apple? Why not? Because they are pure foods that don't contain addictive components and weirdly-spelt unfamiliar man-made ingredients. These ingredients are not added for your benefit, but for the manufacturer's profit margin – mostly to add longer shelf life and a more addictive taste.

- Ultra processed and junk foods are proven to be linked to diabetes, cancer, heart issues and many more auto immune conditions.

- Clearing your diet from these foods will initially cause a detox experience which will feel like the worst hangover or the worst breakup you've ever had. For some, the addiction to these foods has been in their system for so long that giving these up could be like giving up heroin, and cause immense stress to the system.

- The best thing you can do is slowly eliminate them from your diet. Start with cutting out the easiest first.

- It takes two weeks to experience noticeable changes, so be patient with yourself.

- Refer to chapter 1, and **be your very own scientist** on this process.

- When challenged by the process, keep yourself busy, and think of the long term goal.

- Don't forget to be the scientist within and always ask, '**What is causing** these feelings, experiences?
- Things rarely just go wrong with your body. Usually, something you are doing – or eating, or not eating, or drinking or not drinking, is causing the problem. Illness isn't just something inexplicable to be fixed by a doctor; Illness is usually your body's warning light system switching on, telling you to do something different.

Chapter 3: Reduce or Cut out white/simple refined sugar

This stuff has no nutritional value whatsoever, YOUR BODY DOES NOT NEED IT. Gain your health back by cutting it out totally.

- Did you know that cancer feeds on white sugar?
- Did you know that in order for **you to digest foods that contain white sugar, calcium is drawn out of your bones**, causing you to develop osteoarthritis?
- I'm sure you all know that sugar is a major factor in causing **Obesity, Heart Disease** and **Diabetes**… if not, take that to heart. **Literally.**
- Did you know that white sugar upsets the body chemistry? When your body needs to digest a Mars bar for instance, it pulls out nutrients within your body to do so, upsetting the natural chemistry within.

- Did you know that sugar suppresses your immune responses? You need to think about this, particularly now that we are living through a pandemic. In order to protect your immunity, it's easier to just cut it out of your diet all together

- **Many people claim they don't take white sugar because they don't add it to their tea or coffee. <u>This is a massive, massive misconception</u>.** Do you drink sodas? Do you eat any packaged foods? Do you eat tinned foods? Do you eat foods that even say 'No Sugar'? That's actually worse, but I will get onto that in another chapter. Sugar is sometimes added to prescribed drugs and drugs you can buy over the counter. Sugar comes under many different names, and you might find several of them hiding in one product: Fructose, Invert Sugar, Corn Syrup, Maltose - there are loads of ways to hide just how much sugar is in something.

- Did you know that many meat packers feed their animals sugar before slaughtering them? This is to improve the flavour and taste of the meat.

- **Sugar is extremely addictive**. Again like ultra processed foods and junk foods, sugar makes you want more. Look back at the previous chapter and consider apples and broccoli again. If you saw them raw, would you salivate, or does the Kit Kat wrapper do something to you?

- One way to know if a product contains a lot of sugar is to **see where in the ingredients list it is**. If it is the third-to-last ingredient, that means the product is probably ok. If it's within the *first* three, then it's mostly sugar. So, be VERY careful!

- **So, what names does sugar come disguised as? Watch out for these ingredients when you buy your groceries. These are cancer causing, addictive substances and by rights should be illegal:**

1. High fructose corn syrup
2. Maltodextrin
3. Sucrose
4. Sucralose
5. Crystaline Fructose
6. Corn syrup
7. Honey (poor quality - Raw is ok)
8. Modified food starch
9. Refiner's syrup
10. Rice syrup solids
11. Sorbitol
12. Aspartame
13. Maltose
14. Invert sugar

Chapter 4: What's LOW in fat is HIGH in something else that is DAMAGING - Cut out low-fat produce, eat more healthy saturated fats.

If you are like me and have tried every diet out there, you have probably switched to low-fat products at some time in the hope to lose the fat. Well, that won't work in the long term…

- Do you remember being on Weight Watchers, Cambridge diet or Slimming World and feeling deprived, even though you had your healthy (so called) balanced meal? If the answer is yes, this is because counting calories and cutting out fat takes away that sense of **satiation.**

- Do you remember feeling satiated after a really good meal? What did that feel like?

- Did you know you can actually lose fat, whilst feeling satiated after every meal?

- **The sense of satiation** comes from **enough good saturated fats and protein.**

- **Cut out anything that tells you on the label it is low in fat, because it probably is high in other fake foods.** I call these ingredients fake foods because our body has trouble digesting them. Particularly ingredients that you can't pronounce.

- Check the back of a low-fat yoghurt, low-fat dressing or low fat cake and see what you can find. Are there ingredients there that you can't pronounce or identify? Are there any of those hidden sugars listed above? Are there more than about eight ingredients?

- If you can't pronounce the ingredients, and sugar in its many forms (check the list from the last chapter) is high on the list, then it's not easily digestible.

- When foods are hard to digest, they use more nutrients and your own body's energy to digest them. This could be **why you also feel lethargic after a bar of chocolate, or packet of crisps, or even a can of soft drink. Initially, you are high with energy from the insulin spike, but then it crashes, and you need more of the drug food you just had.**

- Eat foods that contain real saturated fats, like avocados, nuts, seeds, 100% whole nut spreads etc. They will fill you and keep you satiated, without any spike or crash. Isn't that what you would like? Oh yes - another point; drizzling salads with extra virgin olive oils but cooking with coconut oil are really good too. Polyunsaturates like Extra Virgin Olive Oil should be eaten cold, as their molecules break apart when heated. But healthy saturate fats like coconut oil should be used for cooking. Try not to use cheap blended trans-fat vegetable oils for this.

- Healthy fats in moderation won't make you fat, but instead keep you satiated and full for longer. They will boost your HDL and reduce your LDL cholesterols.

Chapter 5: The time that you eat matters to you, as do the conditions of digestion

We are all different; this depends on your body clock, your job, and how active you are. To do this, refer to the first chapter on being your own scientist and experiment by journaling your journey. There are some ground rules involved:

- Make sure you have **a gap of an absolute minimum of 3 hours** (try for 4 or 4 and a half) between your last mealtime and sleep (that includes snacks). However, when I did my yoga teacher training in India, our teacher told us that for best digestion after food, one should lay down on their **left side**, to promote digestion. This does work, but in order to lay down, one has to lower themselves to being horizontal - and that in itself is *not* good for digestion. **Again, be your own scientist and experiment.**

- Laying down less than 3 hours or so after eating causes heartburn, digestive issues and trapped wind and can lead to long term issues like Acid reflux and Barrett's Oesophagus

- Some people need to eat breakfast, others don't. Personally, I like to get my yoga and workout in before I have brunch. That's what works for me. But others work far better if they have breakfast.

- Some people skip lunch and eat a heavy brunch, like I do. Others have from 3 to 5 meals a day. The more frequent your meals are (so long as they are small), the faster your metabolism will work as a rule. Again, experiment with this.

- The trick is, **eat when you are hungry and make sure you are satiated but not too full**. Always leave room. It takes 20 minutes to digest water, and the same amount of time for the body to realize it is full. Wait 20 minutes before going for a second helping.

- If you are a meat eater, make sure you eat with at least 4 hours to spare before bed time. If you are a vegetarian or vegan, 3 hours should be ok.

- **Make sure that you are not rushed when eating**. When you are calm, the food digests easier.

- We digest our emotions when we eat, so make sure you say a little something, like grace (prayer) or express a feeling of gratitude before food. This helps massively in raising our vibrations and therefore when the food enters our body, it heals us instead of making us feel bad.

- I like having easy listening jazz in the background to aid my digestion. It creates a calm atmosphere.

- **Make sure that you take a few deep breaths before your first bite.**

- Avoid eating on the go, as your mind and body are in dissonance here. Are you eating or are you moving?

- When you eat, sit down, smell your food, taste your food, chew many times and enjoy the whole process.

- On that note, I am about to have my dinner, so Bon Appetit….

Chapter 6: Cook your own food as often as you can.

We live in a time where almost every meal is pre-ordered. Some of us don't even know what food looks like in its raw state. Shameful! Here are some reasons why you should cook your own food:

- **You know precisely what you put in your meal.** You have control. No extra additives that need not be there.

- When we cook our own food, we add our own love, energy… frustrations maybe? But what we do is all ours. These emotions are heartfelt and real. When we create something authentic through this, there are a lot of positive vibrations that enter our food. These do something positive to us. This may come across a little woo-woo, but we all know there is a massive sense of achievement by even throwing our own ingredients in a salad bowl. It has been prepared by our very own hands and has our love in what we make. We then consume that, knowing what we put in. That's got to be good.

- **When you cook your own food, you can smell and taste the foods. This opens up the senses to the digestive juices, which are then getting ready to receive the food.** This means, when you digest your own cooking, your digestive system does not have to work as hard as it would need to if you were eating some take-away or something at a restaurant.

- The act of cooking in itself, especially when you get used to doing more and more can take away an appetite, and you will only eat what you are hungry for - hence NOT overeating.

- The act of cooking and washing up is also very physical. So guess what? It's like a workout in itself.

- Batch cooking is great - you only need to do the deed once a week and store the remaining 7 dishes in the freezer, to reheat in the week. This means you don't need to agonise over what you will be eating for those meals. They are pre-made for you. How cool is that?

- If you don't have one, get yourself a **slow-cooker.** These are amazing. Before the pandemic, and when I used to go to work, I would cut up some veg, beans and quinoa, then add some veg stock and seasoning. Whilst I was at work and attending my Bikram yoga class 7-9 hours later, it was cooking nicely. When I got back, guess what? My apartment smelt like a home cooked meal that was all ready for me to dig into. And it was! All I had to do was dish out my portion, keep the rest in store for another time. It was *that* easy. Cutting up the veg takes less than 2 minutes, and you can do it the night before. All you do is bung it in the pot before going to work, add water, veg stock, seasoning, and leave it on 'low' heat all day – and it does the rest for you. If you are a meat eater, you'll find that this makes the tastiest meat meals you can imagine as the meat is fully tenderised and the flavours seep fully into the veg. NEVER USE READY MADE SAUCES. These are usually full of unhealthy ingredients.

- Once you get used to cooking more and more, the whole idea of eating out/eating take away will feel less and less appealing. You will get more excited about finding new recipes to try.
- The great thing about cooking at home is the chance to play your up tempo 'Funky Music' and dance, sing and have fun whilst you cook. I love some Abba. What do you dance to?
- It's a great stress reliever too.
- Not to mention that you will be a confident host to future house parties!

Chapter 7: Switch to Plant based food

I am not trying to be a hippy yogic vegan here, but I know that overall, my health has been good and my weight has been well-balanced since switching to plant based foods. Here are some reasons why you should seriously consider the switch:

- Animal protein is more fattening and can contain high amounts of LDL cholesterol. It's therefore bad for the heart too.

- Animal protein, whether it's dairy, meat, or even fish, has hormones, antibiotics and components within that affect our bodies negatively. If you watch 'Seaspiracy', you will see the amount of **micro-plastics** (particles often too small to see) **that are now found in fish.** These plastics go directly into your body when you eat fish. This causes weight gain and contributes to autoimmune conditions like diabetes, cancer, heart disease, eczema as well as asthma and much, much more.

- It's not good for the planet. The way we farm today is raping the world we live in - I'm not mincing my words because in some ways this is actually an understatement. Watch 'Cowspiracy' just to get an idea of what I mean. If we lived in a planet where we fished our own fish from a private river and were able to hand- rear our own cattle using our own home grown feed, it wouldn't be so bad. **But think about how much space that would take for every single person now living in the world** – pretty much all the remaining wilderness, including rainforest, would be used up, which in turn directly contributes to melting the ice caps... There is really not enough space here for me to go on about this, but I think you get my point. Putting animal rights aside, it's simply not sustainable for us humans anymore.

- When we take in stuff that is bad karma, (whatever your belief system is) it will give bad karma straight back to you. So if you eat meat or dairy, think about how the animals were slaughtered and processed, consider how dairy was forcibly taken from them. I know in India, dairy is not so bad because cows are treated with respect there. Think carefully about the journey of your food before purchasing or buying meat or dairy. We are all responsible for our own plate. Artificial insemination and the trauma of tearing calves from their mothers after birth are just two reasons to not support factory farming, but organic farming means relying on the label to tell the truth - and it's simply unsustainable for 7 billion people.

- You won't have to worry about food poisoning! There is no worry about how long the meat has been stored etc. Reheating poultry or meat can be dangerous; all my cases of food poisoning happened when I consumed meat and dairy.

- Digestion will be so much easier without meat or dairy being processed through your gut.

- Your faeces will simply smell, rather than stink. Not to mention bowel motions are much easier when eating plant based (providing you keep up your water intake and eat plenty of veg and fruit).
- You will have more energy about yourself.
- You won't feel the afternoon sleepy feeling that you get from consuming animal protein
- Some plant based foods have a lot of protein - we don't need animals for that. Just look at the elephant, a very strong vegetarian. Where does it get its protein? From plants. **The belief that eating strong animals makes us strong is actually nothing more than 'sympathetic magic'** i.e. similar to painting a tattoo of a bull on your forehead, imagining it makes you strong – something ancient peoples did a long time ago but which has very little basis in science.

So, if you would like to make the switch, I do recommend either: doing a juicing detox program to clean your system first and then switch, **or** slowly switch over by taking some meat out in the first week, and then some dairy, and so on.

The best way to do it right is to see a nutritionist to get your balanced nutritional profile made just for you. My partner Ed Lloyd (on Facebook) is a Plant Based nutritionist. He has been helping many people with the switch over. Look him up.

Chapter 8: Get more protein in your diet

You are probably thinking; now, *that's* a contradiction. You've just told us to go 'Plant Based,' and now you want us to eat protein? Here's what I mean.

- Plant protein is easy to find in mixed foods like beans with rice, quinoa, even baked beans on toast. The formula is: **beans or lentils** combined with **wholewheat pasta, rice or wholemeal bread**. Together, these make a complete protein. Basically, it's **beans + a grain**. So, now, you can get creative. The Indian Kechari dish is a complete protein.

- You can also up your protein by having smoothies with vegan protein powder added.

- Nut butters too are filling. Spread on fruit slices they make a sweet, yet satiating snack.

- The more protein you have, the fuller you will feel, and will snack a lot less.

Chapter 9: 200g of greens on the side of every meal

You are probably thinking, I already have loads of veg already, but *do you?*

- Even if you have loads of veg, they may not be green, and greens act as a cleaning brush to your system.
- 200g of greens on the side will also keep you more satiated
- They can be steamed, boiled or shallow fried greens. Any of your choice.
- About 75% of our plate should consist of veg, and some of it should be all the colours of the rainbow such as carrots, bell peppers, aubergines etc. So add another portion of 200g of greens to keep you satiated and healthy.

Chapter 10: Start your day with a bowl of oats

Who said oats had to be boring? There are so many ways you can do your oats.

- Oats are slow-releasing carbs that create a sense of satiation within the body. They keep you going through the day, without feeling hungry.

- Get creative with oats. Here are some of my own recipes:

1. **Katrina's home made porridge -** oats cooked in water with goji berries, nuts, seeds, raisins, peanut butter (100% whole), Himalayan pink salts and maple syrup (maple syrup is anti inflammatory)

2. My favourite, **Chocolate porridge** - oats, cacao powder, chocolate vegan protein powder, nuts, seeds, raisins, peanut butter (100%). Mix the water in to all the dry ingredients. When it's about ready, stir in the peanut butter. You can actually sprinkle some cinnamon on top, which stabilises insulin. If your protein powder is sweet enough, which they usually are, I wouldn't add any sweetener.

3. **Cabbage porridge -** This is a savoury dish. Chop up the cabbage/red cabbage/savoy cabbage into slices. Chop up half an apple then add some raisins (not too many) and a variety of nuts. All of this goes into the pan of coconut oil. Lightly sauté till a little brown. Then add water to cover and simmer for 3-4 mins on low heat. Now add in a handful or more of oats; it depends on how much

you want. If you have pea protein powder, you can use it as a thickener here. If not, peanut butter is really good too. (I am quite naughty and like a bit of both). When it is thick, it is ready to serve. Again, I like to sprinkle some salt and cinnamon powder on top.

4. You can probably come up with your own form of porridge too. Experiment. Oats for me have taken the place of rice, as rice gives you a false sense of fullness, particularly white rice.

Chapter 11: If you are full from breakfast, forget lunch.

If you have tried my oats for breakfast, it is likely that you will not need lunch. Instead:

- Make yourself a healthy smoothie.
- Have your 200g of greens (if you want to perk your health up) - you could have them with gluten free crackers and marmite on the side. This provides your B12 as a vegan.
- Make yourself a nice cup of cacao powder and almond milk (Hot or cold).
- Have an apple/banana with 100% peanut butter spread.
- Juice yourself carrots, apple, ginger, lemon, and sweet potato. This is filling and full of energy. If you like,

sprinkle a little Spirulina on top with maybe some pumpkin seeds...yum yum.

- If you aren't hungry, keep drinking water through the day.

Chapter 12: Make sure dinner is a complete balanced meal, but not too big.

If you have missed lunch, chances are you will be hungry for dinner!

- **Steam some quinoa** that you can then **fry up** instead of using rice, and add garlic, veg and beans. Beans/ lentils are a great source of protein. **Quinoa on its own also makes a complete protein.** Don't forget the 200g of greens.

- **Grate some cauliflower** into small rice sized grains. Make sure you have enough to shallow fry with garlic, ginger, maybe Tamari soy sauce. You can also steam or stir-fry your veg and beans. Remember, add the 200g of greens on the side.

- Use a **slow cooker to perhaps cook up a bean stew** with veg. This is easy. Just chop up the veg of your choice. Maybe add some Tomato Passata and minced garlic and basil to flavour. Leave it to cook on low heat for 6-8 hours. Meanwhile, before you serve your bean stew, slice some sweet potatoes into wedges - **celeriac chips** are also lovely and can be sprinkled with salt and vinegar for extra flavour. Just chop up a celeriac into slices and marinate them in garlic salts, olive oil an Italian herbs of choice. Place them in the oven or, even better, an **air-fryer/dry fryer** to bake. I have an air fryer/dry fryer that takes just 20-30mins to cook most things that often take longer in an oven. Also, there is no need to pre-heat it.

- There are so many more recipes. These are just some ideas I threw together and they work for me. Basically cutting out animal proteins means you can **eat more, feel more satiated and not get fat.**
- Don't forget to add your **200g of greens** on the side.

Chapter 13: Avoid eating after dinner

Now, this may be a hard one for some of you, but it truly is a good habit to get into. You won't regret it.

- Your body is using a lot of energy to digest its most complete meal of the day. Digesting food is actually one of the most energy-absorbing tasks we do.
- Give your body a break so it can do the work it needs to.
- Anything sweet on top of savoury is not good for digestion, especially eating sweet after/before eating meat. The body uses different methods of breaking

down meat (acids) and starch (alkali) so it will make the job take longer.

- If you are one of these people who are weaning themselves off of sweets after meals, maybe have some pineapple or cacao powder and almond milk as a substitute.

- Fat loss and healing happens well if using this time of fasting between your last meal that night and your first meal the following day.

Chapter 14: But, I want to eat a light breakfast….

That's fine. If you are used to eating your first meal light, do so. But make sure that it is not dairy, and not the usual high sugar/simple carbs like most processed cereals. These things actually *don't* set you up for the day, contrary to the claims on the box: instead, the sugars in them start you on an insulin rollercoaster ride which will push you to have more sugary snacks and drinks later, and generally be hungrier. (Pure oats are the glorious exception as they are complex carbs, don't give you a big insulin spike and their energy lasts for much of the day. But don't go for the processed, instant types with stuff added. Oats are best just as they are).

- Have a **smoothie with vegan protein powder** and your choice of filling.
- Add some Spirulina, Chia, Flax, Chlorella, Matcha or Wheatgrass to your fruit with seeds. The fats from the seeds will satiate you. These are all superfoods with so many vitamins, minerals etc. It's good to start the day eating this way. Chia and Flax contain high amounts of Omega 3.

- Make a juice. There are several ingredients to choose from. These are my go-to snacks:

For a **Green juice**, go for Spinach, Kale, lemon, green apple, ginger, celery/cucumber

For a **Carrot-based juice**, go for 4 carrots, 1 lemon, 1 thumb sized ginger, 3 celery stalks and 2 red apples. You can add a sweet potato or beetroot for more richness. You can sprinkle some of the superfoods mentioned above on top.

- An Oat tracker bar, made in advance. You could stir oats, goji berries, chia seeds, linseeds into a bowl with coconut oil. Then place them in a baking tray into bar sizes of your choice. Wrap them with grease proof paper, place in freezer for an hour, then refrigerate. There you have a tracker energy bar to take with you on the go. You could have this with a Green tea.

Chapter 15: Ok, but lighter breakfasts means I need a substantial lunch.

Yes, it does. So here are a few options:

- Choose one of the oat porridge breakfast options
- Choose one of the dinner options
- Beans on toast is good for a quick fix, it's actually a complete protein. But go for gluten free bread - easier to digest. Also, don't forget the rule of 200g of

greens on the side. If you've never had beans on toast with greens before, try it! You could sauté the greens in some garlic and herbs to complement the tomato sauce. (Also try adding lightly fried onions, mushrooms and tomato halves in first, then the beans later to make it richer in flavour. Sprinkle with black pepper).

- Sweet potato wedges, beans with mixed veg and quinoa. Cook with whatever seasoning you wish.

- Cook in coconut oil. The saturated fat is, paradoxically, better for fat loss than Canola oil or other cheap plant oils. If you can't stand the taste, go for ordinary olive oil (not the Extra Virgin, that's for cold use only).

- Experiment with other dishes. Get creative.

Chapter 16: Can I have a light dinner?

Yes, of course you can. Here are some options:

- Choose from the breakfast or lunch variety

- Blend soup: lightly fry and then stew any veg of choice in a hot pot with veg stock of choice, then blend to texture desired. Aubergine is a good one for thickening stews when it breaks down, but make sure it has been sautéed first.

- Smoothies

- Juices
- Almond and cacao powder
- Use wholewheat pasta or wild/wholegrain rice, which is gluten free. Avoid white rice, white pasta and all shop-style bread – much of it has sugar added. If you really want bread, get gluten free or wholewheat and get it from a bakery if you can. Avoid ALL shelf bread: it has lots of additives to keep it fresh and **often contains sugar** (yes, even brown wholewheat loaves do – check the ingredients, you'll be surprised. Don't forget sugar can appear in other guises too).
- **Limit carbs.** The evening meal for most people is the last big task you'll do in the day – usually people relax after it for a few hours then go to bed. Unless you plan to go out, do something strenuous or active after your evening meal, **do NOT have carbs with it**. You will not burn them off, and so they will simply make you fatter *and* make you hungry just before bed (that's the insulin spike again). This is the other reason not to have desserts, because the spike they give you will likely make you hungry again before bed, not to mention put weight on!
- Maybe the leftovers of any breakfast or lunch?

Chapter 17: Can I have any treats?

The answer is, yes you can - but they MUST not be processed. You can process them yourself. Here are some ideas:

- **Make your own chocolate to refrigerate**. Cacao powder and Extra virgin coconut oil are the main ingredients. You can add nuts, seeds, protein powder, nut butters or even the zest of orange skin (to get that 'Terry's chocolate orange' flavour – Brits will know what I mean). Mix them all in a bowl, add some raw honey/stevia/molasses/rapadura and also some Himalayan pink salts to sharpen the taste. Trust me, the added salt makes it irresistible! Place the mix on a tray and refrigerate for a few hours. It's best kept overnight before sampling. When it's set, cut yourself a piece of your very own chocolate. Watch out – it can be a little addictive, but not nearly as addictive as store bought chocolate and it contains far healthier ingredients.

- **Make your own veg crisps**. Finely slice up carrots, potatoes, sweet potatoes, parsnips, courgettes, aubergines, beetroots and anything else you can think of (although root veg are best). Then drizzle with apple cider vinegar (ACV), salt and whatever other seasonings you wish. Place them on the oven tray or in an air-fryer/dry-fryer and bake for 15-20mins. If your air-fryer has a crisper/fry setting, use that for the last 5-10 minutes to crisp them up.

- **Chick pea snacks**. This is basically the same method as the veg crips/chips above. These are quite nice smeared liberally with Miso paste or Marmite and Apple Cider Vinegar. Nice and crunchy coating with a soft texture inside. Great protein snack. (Don't cook them for too long, though, or they become like bullets and can be hard on the teeth! Experiment.)

- **Sweet potato Chocolate Brownies** - These are my all time favourite. This is a great way to get my Omega 3, Vitamin C and especially Vitamin A levels up. Boil and mash the sweet potatoes, mix them with Extra virgin coconut oil, pumpkin seed, chia seeds, goji berries, vegan protein powder, maple syrup (if not sweet enough) and some Himalayan pink salts to taste. Mix the ingredients then place in a cake tray in the fridge. Have a couple of chunks as your daily omega 3 and protein.

- **Apple, pear or banana dipped with 100% peanut butter** and a dash or cinnamon spread.

- **Nori seaweed wrap sheets.** - You can lightly salt them and add ACV to them too. Have them on their own, or wrap grated cucumber, carrots, beetroots with ACV and Olive oil dressing. By the way, these are a great way to add a seafood flavour to something vegan.

- **3 Medjool dates**
- **1/2 a small cup of mixed nuts, seeds, dried fruit**

- I'm sure you have more ideas. These are to get you started. As you can see, these snacks are filling, satiating, made from real foods and therefore digestible. When foods are digestible, we can eat more of them and not get fat.

- Processed and especially low-fat foods contain ingredients that are not easy digestible. This means the body does not know what to do with them and turns them into excess weight that we don't want. Thus, 'low fat' does not always mean you will lose fat: Processed low-fat products like margarine have only been around since the 1960s and yet obesity has soared since then!

- Make sure your snack is higher in protein and healthy saturated fats than it is in carbs.

- You can snack twice a day or more if you are hungry.

- Make a point to constructively snack, instead of just grabbing what you fancy eating.

- Place your snack on a plate and treat it like a meal.

- Eat it guilt free and enjoy!

Chapter 18: How often should I eat?

If you are genuinely hungry, eat. But, how do I know if I am hungry? Well, here are a few tips to find out.

- Drink a glass of water 30 minutes before eating a meal or snacking. It takes about 30 minutes for water to digest. See how you are feeling after 30 mins - then eat, or don't. Often we think we are hungry when we are actually thirsty.

- If you have followed some of the recommended recipes, cut out ultra processed foods, junk foods and white sugar and then it is highly unlikely you will be hungry for snacks.

- Ask yourself: **'Am I bored, or am I hungry?'** - Try and differentiate between the two. Refer to chapter 1 here. **Be your own scientist.**

- **Get out of the habit of watching TV whilst eating.** This often leads to an uncertainty of emotions and you may just be eating because that's what you are used to doing. And don't ever eat just *because* you are watching TV.

- If you want to snack on chips or popcorn, separate the activity from watching TV. (I know this one is tough!). It doesn't mean you can't on special occasions, but don't make it a habit that you usually do.

- When we watch TV or even read whilst eating, our brain is trying to process two different activities. We need most of our energy for digesting food. So, guess what? When you eat while watching or even reading, you are interrupting the process of digestion and borrowing the energy for something else.
- With all of the rules above followed, listen to your gut. Eat when you are genuinely hungry.
- When you are genuinely hungry, make yourself a rich, protein-filled snack or meal. Every snack and meal you have should contain some form of healthy protein, as this will kill your cravings.
- Feel satiated
- Wait 20 minutes, have a glass of water
- You should feel full after that.
- Keep busy.

Chapter 19: What about alcohol?

Alcohol interferes with the digestive system and liver function, not to mention pretty much everything else. In short, you shouldn't drink, but that wouldn't be fun (socially) would it? Here are some ideas:

- Try to switch to **sulphate-free wines.** Sulphates can cause a lot of headaches and sinus issues as well as inflammation. Usually organic is better, but check the back of the bottle.

- Try to make a drink last the whole night, whatever it is.

- Sip, do NOT gulp, even with beer.

- Maybe change the mindset behind drinking. See who wins holding their drink longer in their hands instead of falling over first. After all, we are trying to make the shift for health.

- Swap your cocktails, alcopops and complex 'brand' drinks to plain wines or straight-up simple spirits (whisky, gin, brandy) instead. Beer is a weight gain cert so best to avoid if you can.

- **Avoid drinking alcohol with ice**. It's really not good for the digestion of alcohol. Have all your alcohol at room temperature. This is one of several reasons why dry red wine and plain spirits are best.

- If you feel you really can't cope with having only one glass, perhaps water it down or have glasses of water between drinks. Make sure you drink water at some point in the evening if consuming alcohol, because alcohol dehydrates you.

- Basically, aim to cut down your alcohol intake altogether.

- Limit going to the pub to once a week, unless you are able to cut out most of the alcohol.

- Perhaps swap it for a hot drink – then you still have a social focus. Many pubs do hot drinks, and tea and coffee are preferable to alcohol! Odd as it sounds, my partner used to start his evening at a local club with a cup of tea in the bar around 10pm, then make his two alcoholic drinks last until around 3am, filling the time in between with fruit juices and soda water… it can be done.

- Another option is to make sure you only stay for one alcoholic drink and not any more.

- If you are a regular drinker, then by limiting alcohol you will find your overall health will improve after a couple of weeks.

- Alcohol ages us very fast.

- **Alcohol calories get used up by the body BEFORE any other calories from a meal.** In practice, this means that if you have a large, three-course meal with alcohol, far more carbs from the meal will get left unused in your system to turn into fat, than if you had it with no alcohol.

- Alcohol causes dehydration, so you must drink at least 2 litres of water after your night out.

- Flush out that stuff afterwards.

Chapter 20: How do I cope with parties and events?

This is a really big one. We are social animals and we need to socialize to some extent for our health. Unfortunately though, in most societies this usually involves food with poor nutrition. Here are some ideas:

- If you host the party/event, then that's easy, just prepare foods that are healthy. There are many real healthy party foods out there. You just have to do some searching.

- If you are going to someone else's do, perhaps eat beforehand, so you don't feel so hungry and will consume less unhealthy food. Also, you will focus more on socializing and not so much on eating!

- The previous option may be seen as rude, and why wouldn't you want to enjoy yourself? In which case, **make an allowance for this event alone**. Super clean up your act as soon as you get back home, such as have an apple and ginger shot juice to clear up those taste buds and bring you back to health. It's dead easy to make: juice 1 apple and about 3-4 inches of ginger (a thumb sized piece). Knock it back as if it was an alcoholic shot; it's far more of a challenge and it will keep you healthy.

- Seriously limit the events you attend unless you are able to exercise control.

- If you struggle with control, perhaps bring your own healthy snacks and foods to the do. Some people with allergies have to live this way. If you think about it, you are allergic to junk food because your body swells up with fat. So, I see that as a form of allergy - I think you get my point.

- Don't obsess about the food: go to the event to meet, to socialise, **the food is not the event**. If it is, then you are possibly going for the wrong reasons.

- Enjoy the company and talk to more people. Keep busy

- When the food is offered, go with your gut instinct.

- Meditate before going, so that your mind is prepared for the challenge ahead.

Chapter 21: Water intake

How much water are you drinking?

- According to some weight-loss companies, you should be drinking roughly 10% your body weight in kg within a day…

- I think that's rather harsh myself, so I go for anything **between 2 litres and 6 litres a day** depending on climate and exertion.

- Most of your water intake should come before breakfast. **Most of it should be actual water, even if you hate it.**

- When you drink lots of water, going for a number two is easier too.

- The best way to drink your first two litres in the morning is to **squat and drink.** The water works its way through your bowels causing you to almost need to go immediately. That way you will have evacuated before breakfast. Wouldn't that feel good? (This is an Indian Ayurvedic method - which I learned during my yoga teacher training).

- Then after your 2 litres, keep a litre of water around you throughout the day. When you feel your mouth is dry, keep sipping.

- Herbal teas, coconut water, juices (home made) are really good through the day to keep hydration up too.

- Dehydration affects moods, causes headaches, dry skin, constipation, nausea and so much more.

- You might be surprised that by drinking a glass of plain water when you feel bad, it will make you feel better. It really does work. If you've had a long, active day out in the sun and are unaccountably irritable, you might put it down to tiredness or too much sun - it's actually dehydration. Drink a couple of litres of water and watch the difference in mood within 20 minutes!

- The body is usually telling you that you need to drink more water when these symptoms arise.
- Don't forget **caffeine dehydrates, as do sodas/soft drinks and alcohol of course.**
- **So, when you have any of these, drink more water to compensate.**
- You should also drink a litre of water after eating ultra processed foods or junk food. Give it 20 minutes though.
- We are often super-dehydrated, and we don't even know it.
- Most of our internal problems would probably be solved by drinking a glass or two of water
- I know the issue for many is needing the toilet, but you are flushing out all these toxins. Not just from what you eat, but from the environment too. If you are at a workplace with toilets, then there really is no excuse – you just need to remember to drink. Log your litres on a small chart or piece of paper. For those on the move, try and drink more just before you arrive at places where there are toilets.

Chapter 22: How much sleep are you getting?

You may not think that sleep is a factor in fat loss, but it is – massively so.

- When you don't sleep, your body can't heal itself making you retain inflammation and pain.

- When you are sluggish, your body will hold on to weight to help it cope with the challenge you are putting it under.

- You need at least **8 hours of undisturbed sleep**

- **Lack of sleep causes stress, which produces more stress hormones such as cortisol. These hormones cause us to retain weight.**

- Your body does not function well when tired. Prolonged tiredness means you are not working at your best capacity. You definitely don't want that.

- You may know what it's like feeling jet-lagged from a longish flight; lack of sleep causes your hormones to be out of whack. **Continuous strain to your body and the fluctuations of hormones could cause the onset of auto-immune conditions such as Hypothyroidism.** This is the thyroid issue that makes it super-easy to gain weight and extremely difficult to lose weight. You certainly don't want that either.

Chapter 23: How much stress are you under?

Did you know that even the stress caused by trying to lose weight can make you retain weight?

- **Over-worrying about anything** causes more production of cortisol, which in turn causes weight gain. So even with all the dieting that you are doing and working super hard to get down to your targeted weight - guess what? **It won't happen (maybe short lived, but not long term), unless you relax about the process you are on.**

- You do have to surrender to the Universe/God or whatever faith or process you are on. Taking everything on yourself causes so much stress that you really do need to unburden your load and take some time out.

- Sometimes stress can cause weight loss, but it often causes weight retention/gain. The body is unpredictable and strange. It's hard to say. This is why you need to **be your own scientist** and measure where you are emotionally.

- **Take time out to walk in nature and get away from technology every day**. Make a point to ditch those devices and be free for a while.

- Dance, shake, move in ways that are unplanned. This clears the clutter in the brain.

Chapter 24: Meditation

What do you do as meditation? We should all do it. These are all different forms of meditation.

- **Meditation is about dropping the ego and tuning into the body**
- **Dance is a form of movement meditation - particularly unplanned improvisational movements.**
- **Singing is a form of vocal meditation.** Allowing your mind to tune into the voice coming out of you in its purest form. Enjoying the sounds you are making with pure pleasure, disregarding everything else.
- **Walking** - Not just walking to the city, but walking alone or with a four-legged companion to the countryside. Take in the air, breathe with purpose. Lose yourself in the sounds of nature, of water and taking in the energies that surround. You will usually feel nourished after this.
- **Swimming** - Not just in a swimming pool, but again also in nature. Feeling the earth/sand/rocks beneath your feet in the water; it's a great form of exchange in energy, is highly invigorating and excellent for physical and mental health. Obviously, do not swim in places where industrial/effluent output, underwater machinery, sluice gates or regular motorboat traffic might injure you. Small, quiet rivers where no motorboat traffic is allowed are excellent. After all, you only need a few feet of water to get in. In the United

States there is a grand tradition of lake-swimming for those who live a long way from the sea. Find local places around you, but if you live within a half-day's drive of the sea then all the better. **Take care** - but the sense of adventure and achievement will do wonders that a swimming pool cannot. It's one of the biggest mood enhancers there is.

- **Shaking** - Spend minutes shaking the whole body intensely, then stand still. Feel the subtle energies within circulate the body. This is your Kundalini, your chi, your energy rising. It is powerful.

- **Sitting meditation** - Focusing on your breath and bringing your mind to your breath. Start with 5 mins and work yourself up to 20 or 30 mins a day. This will set you up nicely.

So these are some of the forms of meditations that you can incorporate into your life to give yourself a fuller and less stressed lifestyle. Enjoy the movement and be at peace with the stillness. This will reduce the stress hormones that cause you to retain weight. If you can do one of these every day, you already have a massive health advantage over many who do not bother. Tip from my partner, Ed: He has worked in a job where on summer mornings, he could go for a natural dip before work in the nearby river and he says he cannot overstate the benefits. Even in the depths of winter, he managed to work in a short 15-25 minute walk in a wood every morning, or wandered across a few fields. He said it is how he coped with 10 years working at the same place!

Chapter 25: Develop your very own Affirmations

A positive mindset goes a long, long way.

- **A positive mind and body go hand in hand, if you want to slim down properly.**
- Say nice things about yourself.
- There are many apps out there that you can download that give you affirmations through the day. Use them and chant them out loud through the day, even if you don't believe it.
- Start making your very own affirmations on how you are changing your life.
- Make this a daily practice.

Chapter 26: How are you feeling?

Every little emotion that comes up about ourselves is valuable information about *you*.

- Did you know **emotions, when stored, can hold on to weight** too? It's called stress (and we know what stress does).
- How we feel affects metabolism because how we feel affects our hormonal balance (particularly in women).

- **Write it down.**
- **Keep a journal.**
- I usually draw columns in my journal and title them: **The Good, The Bad and The Ugly**. That works for me. Whatever system you come up with is personal to your own journey in life.
- When we write down our emotions, they are no longer traumatising us in our brain.
- Not typing, **but writing.**
- When you are done writing, take a deep breath in, and sigh it all away.

Chapter 27a: Move around more

More and more studies are linking obesity to not just excess junk food, but to **not enough movement.**

- I don't mean going to the gym for a full blown 2 hour sesh.
- **Walk around more**
- **Crawl about more** – we don't often crawl as adults
- Move in more unpredictable ways
- Ed and I have dinner on the floor now, picnic style, and we move about more. It helps with digestion too

- **As soon as you have reached 20 mins seated, move**
- Make more herbal tea. Drinking more makes us go to the toilet more – and that's more movement.
- **These regular movements keep you burning fat, without much effort.**
- **They keep you agile and fit and ready to move when you need to.**
- You will creak less and your joints won't be so bad in old age.
- Read **Dan Millman - The Peaceful Warrior**, this explains how it's the little regular movements that matter more to keep us fit, healthy and agile. In my mind, that means slim too.
- Just move about more.

Chapter 27b: Why working out super hard at the gym does not work for everyone

It only works if your heart is in it. If you are not competitive by nature, then the gym is probably not for you.

- I used to be a member at many gyms, and they all left me feeling frustrated.

- I never got into shape even though I worked super hard and had a personal trainer - I spent hours in the gym, to little effect.
- I felt I benefitted more from attending classes and swimming in the pool.
- The noise can be too much for some, over-stimulating the senses. This can make you feel stressed and hurried without even realising it. It induces a competitive, stressy vibe, and that does not help you lose weight.
- There is too much stimulus from others.
- Too many other unhelpful distractions, such as people posing for their pictures by the mirror
- Too much ego flying around!
- For me, I found it hard to get into the right mindset with so much distraction (sound of machines, different TV sets, loud pop music, phones going off, too much chatter). Overall, the ambience brought my mood down, so I knew it was not for me.

Chapter 28: Take up an active class

It's much more fun to learn in a class.

- Perhaps take up martial arts
- Dance
- Workout Zumba or other Aerobics

- HIIT (High Intensity Interval Training)
- Pole fitness
- Belly dance
- Bikram yoga
- Other Yoga types
- Hobbies??
- Anything that takes your mind off your journey and gets it to focus on something you would love to learn and enjoy with others.
- Now, you can do this online too.
- However, be aware how fatigued you may get after some of these classes. For instance, Bikram yoga is a 90 minute Hatha yoga class in a very hot room, roughly 42 degrees C (107 degrees Fahrenheit). I know that I spent most of my afternoon asleep after a Bikram class! So, be aware of how you feel. If you feel lacking energy the next day, *take it easy*.
- Classes may be fun, but focus on how you are feeling the following day.

Chapter 29: Do some HIIT and Body Conditioning

You don't need a gym to do this.

- You just need 30 mins max…
- A yoga mat…

- Access to Youtube…
- Look for a suitable 7 minute workout - That will be your HIIT…
- Then follow on with some Vinyasa Yoga flows - Look for a 20 minute Hatha Yoga flow class.
- Do the above 3-4 times a week - That's your workout.
- The HIIT will help you burn fat and keep you burning for up to 48 hours after the workout. It's only 7 minutes so mentally, you can do this.
- The 20 minute Body conditioning through yoga will tone your whole body, whilst clearing your mind as well. The nature of yoga ends with gratitude and corpse pose – it is a great way to begin your day.

Chapter 30: Less is more sometimes

Less can be more sometimes when it comes to workouts:

- **Your body needs time to heal**, so it can feel strong when you push it next time.
- Proper rest is just as important, or if not even more than the exercise you do. Let your body feel properly rested before attempting another workout.
- **Give it a day or two between sessions**
- **If you fancy more, then walk more, move more**.

- On days that you don't do HIIT/body conditioning/ an active class, perhaps do an activity with more Yin energy like Tai Chi, Yin yoga (restorative yoga), walking or light swimming.

- When we do more than our body and mind are ready for, it can cause inflammation and, surprise surprise - you got it, you retain fat. You don't want that. Again, it's stress on the body.

- Listen to your body; **if it's tired, don't push.**

- **Our metabolism works based on calories in and out, but also a BIG part of that is hormonal. If you are too tired, you are putting your body under more strain.**

- This book is about staying slim for life. We are not on a fix-it-quick mission here.

- **This has to be sustainable.**

Chapter 31: Have a day off from it all

Take a break.

- When I was studying for my yoga teacher training in India, every day apart from Sunday was designated for meditation and yoga. We had one day to ourselves. That day, we didn't even meditate. I actually craved some pure consumerist capitalism and so I watched 'Friends' or 'Sex and the City', just to feel a bit less spiritual! Basically, I just needed the break.

- Even take a break from the journaling, unless you don't want to.
- **At least once a week, don't plan that day - just see what happens instead.**
- That day could be the day assigned to a picnic, walk in nature or swim.
- Maybe that day could be your movie night, where you do actually allow yourself the rare treat of popcorn with a movie.
- **It's about having some form of balance. Make sure you don't have a day/night off every night.**

Chapter 32: When you indulge, enjoy it!

When you have a party, eat out, indulge, enjoy it!

- That's right, you will be back to normality the following day, so make the most of it.
- Enjoy your indulgence, GUILT FREE.
- When we feel **guilty**, we feel shame, and with that comes stress and… you know what that brings? That's right, **weight gain.** You don't want that. So, enjoy your food, for life is short. Just don't go mad or life will be shorter ☺☺☺

- As long as you keep your indulgence to a max of **once every 2 weeks** or even less often, you won't do yourself any lasting harm.
- Obviously the less indulgent you are, the better it is for you.
- However, once you decide to indulge, do it whole heartedly.
- No regrets.

Chapter 33: Ditch those weighing scales

Weighing scales are the object of all weight watchers' unhappiness, so *why weigh?*

- What is weighing yourself regularly really going to do? Be honest. You say it's for you to keep an eye on yourself so you don't gain too much weight, but **does it actually do that?**
- People who weigh themselves regularly have reported a great amount of depression connected to their weight. Guess what depression does? It makes you retain weight.
- Weighing scales cause necessary stress. In fact, **in Anorexia Nervosa, the urge to weight oneself is viewed clinically as no different than the urge to light up for smokers, or to drink for alcoholics, or to binge for binge-eaters. It is an addictive behaviour.**

- **Muscle is much heavier than fat.**
- You could be retaining water, especially if you've just drunk 1 litre or more.
- **Throughout the day, our weight fluctuates.**
- **You won't know your true weight until several days after your indulgence anyway. It doesn't show the next day, like you think.**
- **You put your happiness on hold just because the numbers go up.**
- Should numbers dictate your happiness, if you were happy beforehand?
- When we are unhappy… yes, the weight goes up.
- So overall, there is no reason to keep weighing scales in the house.
- Instead, look at yourself in the mirror.
- Take pictures of yourself.
- Use the 'trousers of truth' to guide you, or another tell-tale garment you want or like to wear.
- Your clothes are more honest than scales.
- How do you feel?
- Are you more energetic?
- **As long as your overall health and wellbeing has improved too, then you are on the right track.**
- Bottom line? Chuck those scales out.

Chapter 34: This is probably the most important thing I will tell you - Educate yourself on the different ways of eating that are out there.

There are so many variations of diets, ways of eating etc, you need to find out what suits you.

- Do you want to go Vegan? Vegan involves not just going plant based but is connected to looking after the planet, protecting animals and so much more than just what you eat. In terms of Diet, being vegan means you don't touch meat, poultry, seafood, dairy and even honey or anything else relating to a living being (including not wearing leather). Most people who claim to be vegan aren't in fact really 100% vegan.

- There are healthy vegans who eat mostly beans, legumes, pulses, grains and veggies

- There are unhealthy vegans who eat mostly processed foods, high in carbs (you don't want that one)

- There is an alternative - **Plant Based - This simply means getting most of your nutrients from foods that are plants. It may mean that 75% - 98% of your food are plant based and the remainder could be dairy, seafood or even meat.**

- You could be Vegetarian - This involves eating similar foods to the vegan or plant based diet, with the added content of dairy.

- There are also have healthy and non healthy vegetarians too. Some will eat more processed foods with high carb content, and others will eat real foods.

- If you do choose to have animal protein in your diet, make sure you limit it to once or twice a week. Doing it more, will retain more fat. We now know that animals have high levels of hormones, antibiotics and much more within them as a result of how they are reared. Also, when they are killed they release high levels of stress hormones. Guess what that does to us? You got it, it helps you gain weight. So, think carefully about that. Meat, before the 20th century, was a luxury item to many (and still is in some parts of the world). **Try and emulate our ancestors that way and keep it a special treat, not an everyday need. You don't need it everyday; we're not designed to be obligate carnivores.**

- **Keto should be done with the guidance of a nutritionist (and <u>Vegan Keto can be very dangerous</u>).**

- **ALL diets that are short-lived are a temporary measure; they will not give you the freedom you wish for**. However, with the support of a nutritionist, you can incorporate them in your lifestyle for a quick boost from time to time. But we are trying to stay away from that.

Chapter 35: Juicing

Juicing is a great boost to your immune system. It can also be used as a reset after a binge or night out.

- **Juicing can be incorporated into your lifestyle at any point.**

- When I have felt that I have had an indulgence, say someone's birthday party or Christmas, I will go on a 3-5 day juice fast.

- There are recommended programs by **Jason Vale** and **Joe Cross**. Do a bit of research of your own with this. Juicing is actually great fun to do.

- **My recommended watch:** *Fat, Sick and Nearly Dead* **by Joe Cross.**

- **My other recommended watch:** *Superjuice Me* **by Jason Vale.**

- I have done both programs and find both are valuable. I even mix the two up sometimes.

- **Find what works for you, and drop the rest.**

- Sometimes if I eat a heavy breakfast, or lunch, I will have a juice for my next meal instead.

- Sometimes I have a juice instead of a protein snack.

- **Juices are amazing energy boosters. They are full of micronutrients and minerals, in quantities we can't get by just eating fruit and veg.**

- Making a juice can take something like: 8 large carrots, 2 apples, 1 lemon, 4 celery stalks, 1 thumb sized root ginger, 1 beetroot and 1 sweet potato. It's not possible to sit down in one meal and eat all of these! But you can imagine the nutrients from the fruits and veggies are really dense.

- **It truly is good to get into the habit of incorporating a juice a day, if at all possible.**

- Sometimes I will have 2 juices and 1 meal a day - especially if I am feeling like I have over eaten recently.

- These are the adaptations you can make to balance overeating when out.

- That's not to say 'keep on overeating' - more to say, be wise about when you overeat and what you do to overcome it.

- You have to do something, or else you will continue to grow bigger, and you really don't want that.

- This is why you should constantly **be your own scientist**. *"Check yourself before you wreck yourself"* - As Mr. Wu from the TV series Benidorm often says during mishaps ☺ Lol… just had to put this one in.

Chapter 36: Fasting

There are so many methods of fasting out there, which one is right for me?

- So, you want to do your own research on this.

- There are religious fasting ways, such as Ramadhan for Muslims. The issue with this is the lack of water, particularly during daylight. That's when we are awake and need to water ourselves more. So please be aware of this. **Lack of water causes dehydration which can bring about other illnesses, chiefly diabetes.** Data in densely Muslim-populated countries shows a high amount of diabetes: poverty aside, I'm not sure if there is a link - but I do know that we need water to survive. Being hot and not being able to drink, and then downing a load of soft drinks, dates or sweets after a fast is really not the healthiest of choices and puts immense strain on the pancreas and kidneys. So, if you do decide to fast this way, then make sure you spend most of your days asleep or indoors. Your body can deal with lack of food, but water is a must.

- Some people do **bread fasts** - where they only eat water and bread. This is all going to turn into sugar and cause a lot of constipation too. So, in terms of health, it's not the best option.

- **A water fast** is where you only consume water for 24 hours and for some, up to 72 hours. This is probably the most powerful fast. You need water, and your body will survive not eating. When it goes without food after 24 hours (some cases are less and some more), the body enters a condition known as **'Autophagy'**. Autophagy is when the body cleans unwanted and damaged cells out of the system. It gives the body the chance to generate new cells. When the body does this, you will experience a sense of being renewed and reborn on a cellular level. Therefore it can correct problems within the body.

- **5:2 fasting diet** - I have done this one. In fact I did it for 2 years non-stop! Yes it works, but when doing it long term, the mind gets annoyed and then the fasting stops working (That was my experience anyway). The 5:2 is where you eat 500 calories a day twice a week for a woman, and 600 calories a day twice a week for a man. The rest of the time you eat normally. This is great initially, and can be done from time to time, like the juicing, when you feel you have indulged.

- **16:8 Intermittent fasting.** This is when you fast for 16 hours (for most of it, you are asleep), and you eat in an 8 hour window. This form of fasting is the most manageable. In fact it's really good. I do this one 1-3 times a week. So I will eat before 5pm, and eat again around noon the following day. I find that this one prevents you from feeling too hungry. But like anything, don't do it every day.

- Do your research, look into all options.
- Find what works and drop the rest.
- Incorporating fasting from time to time is good for the system, so **don't see it as a diet, it is a detox** - just like the juicing.

Chapter 37: Films/Programs to watch

These are a MUST watch if you want to re-educate your brain to what's really going on.

- Gamechanger - Netflix
- Cowspiracy - Netflix
- Seaspiracy - Netflix
- A Plastic Ocean - Netflix
- What the Health - Netflix
- Michael Mosley on the 5:2 Fasting diet (You may want to do some researching on Google and Youtube). There are articles and websites, the initial program doesn't appear to be there on Youtube.
- Fat, Sick and Nearly Dead by Joe Cross - Netflix/Youtube
- Superjuice Me by Jason Vale - Youtube
- There are probably more out there. Keep updating yourselves with the latest findings over nutrition, the planet and what is best for you.
- Please be aware what is good for the planet is also what we need, because it needs to be sustainable.
- The way I see it, our health is important, as is the health of others around us and the health of the planet. Well - actually I put the planet first, as we

only have one Planet Earth! So, that for me has to be a driving force in what I choose to eat.

- So yes, if you dive deeper you may find political issues with Avocados for instance. I won't go into that, but you have to do your own research, **be your own scientist** and be awake and alert in your own journey. Be interested, or else it won't work.

Chapter 38: This is a different way of being

You are now a conscious human on a mission to solve your health whilst making sure there isn't a big carbon footprint on the planet.

- When we look at our journey as holistic, it makes sense.
- Collectively as a society, we have a moral obligation to our home - Planet Earth.
- Whatever we buy, WE are responsible.
- **It seems to make sense that in order to protect the environment and do the right thing, a big part of it is about switching to plant based foods.**
- So, by doing so, you will be cutting out a heck of a lot of the stuff that makes you fat.
- So double whammy there. **The planet and your health taken care of.**

- You have to feel proud and good about what you are doing, to keep yourself motivated.
- **Take an interest in your own development.**
- Study, research, plan and find ways of improving your carbon foot print, by also taking care of your health too.
- **You can allow for mishaps, for occasional treats that are not normally how you eat, but don't let it crawl into the next day.**
- **One day is fine, your body can cope with that. In fact, a change is good (even if it is negative, from time to time, so the body still remembers what it was like to eat that junk).** My partner Ed calls it 'throwing your body the occasional curve ball.' Otherwise it gets complacent.
- So, if you know you ate junk one day, correct it immediately on the next meal.
- You have the tools in previous chapters to help you.
- Don't be so stringent, yet be strong with yourself too.
- You deserve health and to be happy.

Chapter 39: Ways that you can make a start

You have all the information in previous chapters to help you so now, how do you start?

- Simple - decide you **want to make a change**

- Use the first week to analyse what you currently eat, by keeping a diary for at least 3 days.

- **Look at what foods you could begin to cut out that may cause inflammation, say, start with cutting out sugars (including all packaged foods that contain sugar and that includes things like bread and cereals) for 2 weeks, then resume sugar and cut wheat for 2 weeks, then go back to wheat and try cutting out dairy for a couple of weeks – see what happens in each case.** If there's still no change, try cutting out meat next. Then try soy products (other than fermented soy), then cruciferous veggies – eventually you should find something that makes a difference when you cut it out.

- Look at the previous chapters and slowly add more veg by reducing the carbs, animal proteins and dairy

- Get yourself a nutritionist to guide you. My partner, Ed Lloyd is a plant based nutritionist and he can help you. Again, look him up on Facebook. He has a Facebook group called 'Let's talk crap', which is all about digestive and bowel issues, which were his motivation to get into healthy eating. Feel free to join the group, as it is free.

- Journal your journey.
- Remember this is **not a diet but a lifestyle shift**, so don't expect quick changes.
- **Cut down/out processed foods and sugar**. This one I can't stress enough.
- Look for alternatives that suit you.
- Add in your 7 minute workout routines 3 times a week
- Move more.
- Stress less.
- Meditate.
- Do more of the stuff you enjoy.
- Watch the recommended programs in the chapter above - that will motivate you.
- You may want to even begin with a juicing fast, as I did to clean my system from animal proteins before I went plant-based - it takes away any taste for meats.
- Journal more and research more.
- **Be your own scientist.**
- **If you need 1:1 guidance, I run tailor made programs, specific to your needs. Look me up, Kundalini with Katrina on Facebook. Feel free to join my Facebook group, Kundalini with Katrina. It is free.**

Chapter 40: The truth about BIG FOOD COMPANIES

From the programs recommended above, you will know that they are:

- Steadily destroying the planet for their own profit.

- Lying to us again and again.

- Poisoning us with addictive components in their food, which isn't actually food but 'food product' i.e. edible advertising. Edible advertising is designed to do one thing; enrich the company that makes it.

- They are linked up with BIG PHARMA – the less healthy you are, the healthier their bank balance is.

- They manipulate us very cleverly with their packaging and marketing.

- BIG FOOD has been part of our lives growing up, so the associations to fun times with families and friends are all mixed in with what they are selling. It's very clever.

- It is pure manipulation.

- They are so BIG, they know they can get away with it.

- **They pretend that they care about the environment and health by sponsoring events and much, much more. They often sponsor research to prove that their food poses no health risks**. This is sadly common. A quick bit of googling can show you which big companies are behind which research. For instance, I have seen firms that sell cakes sponsoring Cancer Awareness events (and thus gaining positive PR). This is basically no different from a protection racket – endangering people and then making profit from their misfortune, or like clubbing someone over the head and then bringing them to hospital whilst posing as their rescuer.

- They are BIG giants that are trying to keep us all sick, so we buy more of their stuff to feel emotionally better when all it is doing is making us feel more and more ill and therefore more dependent on them. It's a vicious circle, and it makes megabucks.

- Be wise, **Escape the Matrix**, the food-diet trap that they want to keep you in.

- **Be your own scientist and resist the packaging**. It's tough, but like a muscle, the more practised you are at resisting it, the better you become and guess what, you're suddenly not as fat as you were.

- Also, be aware that the plastic packaging may have dangerous chemicals in them, such as BPA. These mess with our hormones.

Chapter 41: The truth about BIG PHARMA

Pretty much the same as BIG FOOD, it's all one.

- Big Pharma are pill pushers…

- Basically, that means drug pushers.
- The side effects of many of these drugs often outweigh what they are supposed to treat, requiring more drugs to treat the side effects of those drugs… and so on.
- If you eat right, you don't need Big Pharma except in emergencies.
- I used to be asthmatic and needed my inhalers every day. Since going plant-based, I no longer suffer with asthma. It's been 6 years since I touched an inhaler. **The nurses keep encouraging me to have one on me**, which I did for a while, until I felt that all I was doing was spending money unnecessarily on a drug I never used. **Deep breathing, yoga and good healthy food cured me.**
- **Statins are being pushed to people who don't even suffer with high cholesterol/high blood pressure, simply because they are of the age that they may encounter high cholesterol/high blood pressure**. This happened to my dad (and to my partner's mum and dad), and in the case of my dad, **he actually had low blood pressure instead!** I helped him clean up his diet and his health has much improved *without statins*. He took them initially and it aged him by 10 years. I told him to stop, and when he did he was looking much healthier. Don't just do something because your doctor tells you, especially if you didn't ask for it; many just want to sell you pills. And more pills to counter the side effects of those pills, and so on.
- Doctors are paid to go on long conferences with BIG PHARMA to learn about the latest drug. I also un-

derstand that doctors are encouraged to sell these drugs to patients, even if they don't need them. By contrast, **doctors (by their own admission) spend less than a few hours (out of 6 years' training!) studying nutrition.**

- **So much is solved by simply drinking a litre of water. Have you had yours yet?**

- **We can solve our health problems with eating right and exercising. We all know this deep down.**

- I am **not** urging you to get off any drugs you are on right now. It is dangerous to do so, and yes, you do need your doctor to monitor your condition.

- What I am saying is that **before you go for a higher dose or a different drug, check your situation first. Am I eating right? Am I drinking enough water? Am I exercising enough? When you know you have tried everything, and it's still persisting, then yes, by all means seek other help. But even then, consider what you are being told. Does it sound right?**

- There is a place for allopathic medicine. For instance if you have appendicitis, or have been in a car crash, then that is what it is there for. **But it is NOT there to prop up an unhealthy lifestyle.**

- **Autoimmune conditions can be avoided through good nutrition and lifestyle.**

- This is all common sense, so make it your responsibility to do your own research and find what works for you and drop the rest.

Chapter 42: We are all different

Just because someone is doing something and it's working for them, does not mean it will work for you.

- Consider your health.
- Do you have thyroid issues?
- Do you have chronic fatigue?
- Do you have other auto-immune conditions?
- Your age, gender, mindset - these all matter.
- Do you like competitive activities?
- Are you like me, where you prefer not to compete because competing gives you bad feelings?
- Do you like to take your time?
- Do you have an excess of energy?
- Do you struggle with having energy?
- All of this affects how we lose, gain and maintain fat.
- **This is where your journaling is important**. You need to know who and indeed *how* you are, and what kind of person you are.
- There are personality tests and behavioral tests online that you can do to help you discover what kind of person you are.

- It took me 7 years to get to the mental and physical space where I am - which I am content with. I know the little shifts I have to make from time to time, as I know I don't like being bigger than I feel I should be naturally. **So, I check myself in terms of how I look and feel - but nothing else.**

- If I look and feel a little larger/more tired than I should, I return to my journal, and see what I can cut out or change and maybe do a juice fast to get me back to where I was - then eat cleanly again.

Chapter 43: What is your TRUTH behind weight/fat loss?

Weight/Fat loss is never good enough a reason by itself to get into shape.

- I have tried diets of all kinds, controlling my eating one way or another for the sake of getting slimmer. What did it do? It initially helped me lose lbs, but after a while, my mind rebelled against the diet and I ate more to compensate. This, I understand, is all too common a pattern.

- The truth is that weight/fat loss was never enough for me. It may not be enough for you if you are like me. Trust me, most people are the same in this.

Once you dig deep enough, you will find the real reason behind your goal is not to see the numbers going down on the scales, but something far more.

- I came to this discovery when I saw how diabetes in my family was causing loss of limbs and frequent strokes. That scared me far more than getting the numbers to go down on the scales!

- When I cleaned up my diet so that I would not get diabetes, not only did I gain more health, but I lost quite a lot of lbs too. My aim was to be way out of the pre-diabetic zone, where I am now, and to be as healthy as I can be, so I don't get strokes or lose any limbs. Having diabetes in both family sides really scares me, and seeing so many members suffer severely with it was my driving force. I was not going to be like them. So, that is my true reason.

- **What is your true reason?**

- You need to get specific.

- You need to start with asking yourself 'What does it mean to me that I need to lose weight?'

- If your answer is, say, because I want to fit in my clothes again, then ask 'What does it mean to me to fit in my clothes?'

- I think you can see where I am going with this. Keep asking yourself, keep digging down until you get to **a truth about you** rather than a generalisation that loads of people come up with.

- You may peel back the onion and eventually come to happiness. This is very common. How does happiness look, what does it feel like? Who are you sharing these moments with?

- Really get clear on this.

- If you need help in this you could always ask a friend to play the role of a coach and coach you through this just by digging deeper and asking you 'What does it mean?' Until you discover your real truth.

- **Your truth may be totally different from what you expect.**

- **Until you find your truth, transformation won't really happen. At least, not a deep meaningful transformation anyway!**

- This is really important.

Chapter 45: What do I do, now that I know my TRUTH?

Now you know your Truth behind fat/weight loss:

- **Mind map** - write everything about your truth that scares you.

- Get very clear why your truth is driving you.

- **Consider what would happen if you did absolutely nothing. Follow that thought through. It's scary, I know, but knowing this will keep you motivated, particularly when times are tough.**

- Write down this truth in as many places as you can around the house.

- Make a plan based on what you have read so far in this book on **how you will start and carry on with this journey.**

Chapter 46: Talk to your friends and family

Let your loved ones know what you are about to do.

- Explain to your loved ones that you are on a transformational journey.
- Share this book with them - if you feel they would understand.
- Have friends and family on board so that you are not only supported, but the chances of you slipping will be less likely.

Chapter 47: Mindful Eating

When we eat, it's very important to enjoy our food.

- Have you paused to consider how you eat?
- It's good to get into the habit of blessing your food before you eat, even if you don't believe in God/gods/Universe or any form of creation. Here's why:

- When we bless our food, we express gratitude before eating.
- Expressing gratitude removes the urgency around eating.
- It creates space and love in the body and mind before taking food in.
- It prevents indigestion.
- It slows down the pace of eating.
- Eating slowly to savour, smell and taste allows the digestive juices to secrete even more so you can digest your meal properly.
- Take time between each bite.
- Enjoy your meal like it is your last meal. **Never rush eating, ever.**
- Make the most of every bite; chew and savour many times before swallowing.
- Avoid drinking (even water) whilst eating. Your body needs to work on digesting the food.
- **Wait 30 minutes before you drink.**
- Remain seated for at least 30 minutes after your meal if you can. Of course you can shift pose to get comfortable, but don't get up from the table.
- **You can sit on your knees as that is excellent for digestion (thunderbolt pose). Much of Asia eats this way, and they have fewer stomach/digestive issues than we have in the West.**
- Express a sense of gratitude after every meal.

Chapter 48: Gratitude

Gratitude keeps away negative emotions.

- Every time we express gratitude, we haven't got space for fear/anxiety.
- These two emotions can't co exist.
- When we feel fear, we are producing more stress hormones that cause us to retain or gain fat.
- Even a little bit of stress can retain fat.
- When we replace fear with gratitude, even faking it, it becomes real.
- So, when you feel fear, write down your fear, then see if you can write the opposite of your fear and capture the emotion of that, e.g. 'I am scared that I don't have enough money to pay for my rental'. The opposite of that is, 'I have a lot of money and I can pay my rental'. Even though this statement doesn't feel true, sit with it, live it, close your eyes to imagine and experience it. This is **manifesting,** and one way or another, you will find a way to make it true. **Let it go.**
- We will explore manifestations in the next chapter.
- Return back to gratitude.

Chapter 49: Manifestation

We are our thoughts.

- What we think, we manifest.

- So, simply put, what you think becomes real.

- You may want to look into **Abraham Hicks - Law of Attraction** or **Teal Swan** on Youtube **explaining how manifestation works.**

- However, there is a trick to manifestation. The more passionate we are about something (good or bad), the more that thing becomes a reality.

- This is why when someone is poor they become poorer. They are attracting more vibrations of what they already have.

- The trick is to put yourself in the place of already receiving what you manifest.

- So, if getting smaller in size is what you want, you need to put a lot of energy into imagining what that will look like, the clothes you are wearing, even the smells of places you may go to.

- For manifestation to work, you need to visualise, get specific and then let it go; as if it's not important and you are just surrendering to the universe.

- If you fear the lack of something (opposite of abundance), you will manifest more of that. I know, I have been there too.

- The only time I was able to manifest being the size I wanted was when I gave up my weighing scales. When the numbers go up, I am asking for more of that, because I passionately feel hate towards the scales. This passion of hate attracted more of it! I had to work super hard - and yet I actually gained more weight.

- **So the trick is, make a note of what you want.**

- **Imagine what that's like.**

- Spend time throughout the day going into your head, seeing exactly what that would look like.

- Then the big thing is, **trust that it is happening.**

- With the trust, you are surrendering and fear is gone, leaving you only gratitude.

- Gratitude vibrates so high that your manifestation is coming true.

- Believe it and don't question the time, as that is a test you don't need to pass.

- **The more you are tested, the more you question, the more you question, the more self doubt there is.**

- Where manifestation is concerned, you kind of have to **switch off your scientific mind**.

- I am where I want to be now: physically, emotionally, mentally and financially (not too bad too)

- **Develop your own mantra from this and say it every time you have self-doubt.**

- Mine is, I'm where I want to be, and I am going where the energy takes me. I am aligned.

Chapter 50: Alignment

In brief: Alignment is everything.

- Alignment is physical, emotional, mental, spiritual and universal. For starters!

- True alignment happens when your body, mind and the universe are one in making a decision.

- You know a decision is in alignment with you and the universe when there is no resistance.

- Resistance takes the form of hold-ups, things going wrong and just bad luck.

- When our bodies are in alignment, our mind becomes more aligned and the choices we make are in alignment with the universe too.

- **You can become aligned by aligning your spine, core and energetic body.**

- The spine can be corrected by a chiropractor (Chinese traditional chiropractor)

- **Do Hatha yoga practice on a regular basis. Working through Vinyasa flows (downward dogs, planks, cobras, and downward dog again) is really good for creating a beautiful, aligned and spacious spine.**

- Regular practice of Chi-Kung, Tai-Chi, Kundalini yoga, Reiki, Sound bowl healing and many more energetic healing methods will help increase the upward-flow of energy that will put the body, mind and emotions in alignment.

- **As a Kundalini yoga teacher, I highly recommend the method of using internal vibrations to release anything stuck within. This opens up so many possibilities, emotionally, physically and universally too.**

- When the body, mind, emotions and the universe that surrounds you are all in alignment, not only are your manifestations achieved faster, but you are healed and can now be of service to others.

- When you are at this place, you never need to follow any regimented way of life. You will automatically know what you need, and what to do.

- **You also no longer need to be the scientist, you can release that and just be.**

- Your body, mind and emotions are as one and whatever you do is not resisting anything, and therefore life is good.

Chapter 51: Kundalini Yoga

There are so many mixed messages about Kundalini Yoga, so let me share my understanding.

- Kundalini yoga is what got me out of a very dark place. I lacked confidence, I was an over-eater, and came from a place of 'lack of…'

- Kundalini yoga involves creating a surge of internal energy from the base of your spine upwards to the crown.
- The practice focuses on chakras (energetic centres - part of the subtle body).
- We have 7 chakras that we focus on.
- Each chakra correlates to emotions, conditions, physical ailments, our behaviours and way of life.
- When energy is able to flow unhindered, our general health and wellbeing is good.
- If not, it's not so good!
- Many of the problems we face can be corrected by simply getting 'unstuck' energetically.
- The practice of Kundalini yoga does this.
- The way I teach is based on *Kundalini Tantra*, which is the Indian traditional method. I also incorporate some of Yogi Bhajan's methods (made popular by several Gurus in America).
- Many practitioners portray Kundalini Yoga to be spiritual, and yes it is – if by 'spiritual', they mean simply that you are aligning your energetic body. The experience can feel somewhat spiritual, as there isn't a physical way to explain the emotional transformation that takes place. But my practice of it is completely secular and scientific.
- It was only when I had completed my studies in Kundalini yoga that I was able to live comfortably and trust that the universe has my back - and that all is well.

- Being able to let go like this prevents stress and helps me stay balanced and healthy in an uncertain world.
- We know what stress does to us, right? It retains fat. So, Kundalini Yoga will unblock you energetically, so you have nothing to worry about and can trust the Universe/God.
- If you need a Kundalini yoga teacher for transformation, look me up on Facebook - Kundalini with Katrina, and I can help you.

Chapter 52: Chi Kung

A traditional Chinese practice to control and manipulate energy both within and outside you.

- The manipulation of energy gives one the sense of control and strength.
- It is calming for the mind, as the body moves with the breath.
- Regular Chi Kung controls fat gain, overall health and wellbeing.
- Having this practice as part of your life at least once a week does so much good.
- You can find online teachers and Youtube videos that are helpful.
- Avoid practicing during menstruation.
- It is best to seek a professional if unsure.

Chapter 53: Vibrational work

Put simply, shaking.

- Shake with the voice.
- Let go of stuck energy.
- We have fat cells; I sometimes imagine that the vibrations burst the cells.
- Maybe they do and maybe they don't, but I always look slimmer after a 15-30 minute shaking body and voice session.
- You don't have to think about it.
- Have your favourite music playing and lose yourself in your own rhythm.
- Shaking is a great way of stimming for those (like those on the Autism Spectrum) who may need to stim.
- Shaking releases the stuff you can't release otherwise.
- I incorporate this method in my Kundalini yoga teaching as it releases trauma.
- **Trauma, stress, anxieties, fears, frustrations and any negative vibes really and truly can be shaken off.** You just have to lose yourself in it.
- Once you finish shaking, stand still, and feel the energies you have stirred up surge within you.
- You can then sit still and meditate on these sensations.

- You can imagine the energies burning off your excess fat.
- Visualise, as I talked about in the chapter on manifestation, and it will help you lose the fat.
- The more intense you shake, the more calories you will be using.

Chapter 54: Walking

I don't just mean walking to the shops or around the house!

- I mean getting your walking boots/shoes on and going out in nature.
- **There is nothing like surrounding yourself with trees to soak up all the negativity that you carry within you.**
- It's a great source for meditation.
- **It gets you away from being stuck indoors and doing computer work.**
- It changes your breathing and oxygen levels.
- **You get to lose yourself in seeing beautiful wildlife, flora and fauna.**
- If you walk by flowing/moving water such as streams, rivers or the sea, the sounds are so relaxing and you can forget your troubles.
- **It's a chance to get connected with nature, with the source of you. We are animals, we come from**

nature, not from office blocks, houses, hospitals or factories; this is the *real* world.

- Nature is real. The man-made stuff that we live in and work in disconnects us from what's real. It's easy to forget that our human world is actually a fake one, and the societal disconnection from the natural world very recent (last 150 years or so). Before that, man lived much more in harmony with nature and the countryside.

- This disconnection causes illness, autoimmune conditions, stress and therefore fat gain.

- Overall, walking is great exercise and it's exactly what we were built to do. Do it.

Chapter 55: Swimming

I don't mean just in a swimming pool.

- **Get out there and swim in the sea, rivers, lakes**, under waterfalls (if you have them).

- Connection with real, fresh running natural water is like nothing else. There's no substitute.

- It washes away your toxins and negative emotions.

- Submerge, but only if the water is clean enough.

- **Cold swimming is highly recommended for your immunity.**

- Obviously, do not swim in places where industrial/effluent output, underwater machinery, sluice gates or regular motorboat traffic might injure you. Small, quiet rivers where no motorboat traffic is allowed are excellent. After all, you only need a few feet of water to get in. In the United States there is a grand tradition of lake-swimming for those who live a long way from the sea. Find local places around you but if you live within a half-day's drive of the sea, then all the better. **Take care** - but the sense of adventure and achievement will do wonders that a swimming pool cannot. It's one of the biggest mood enhancers there is.

- Swimming in cold water increases serotonin levels, which elevates mood.

- When your mood is up, manifestation is up, vibrations are up and what you want in life is easier to achieve.

- Overall, swimming is fantastic exercise that does not put pressure on any parts of the body.

- I recommend doing this weekly or more. **Remember to follow the warning guidelines above.**

Chapter 56: Avoid busy places

I know this can be rather tricky, because at some point or another, you just can't!

- **When possible, stay away from busy places.**
- They soak up your positive vibes and fill you with so much energetic confusion.

- People from all walks of life have different vibrations causing you (if you are like me and are susceptible to it) a lot of headaches, emotional pain etc.

- When we surround ourselves by too much frantic energy, it messes with our own system and prevents us from tuning in with our minds and bodies.

- Also, avoid family/friendship/relationship drama, i.e. all emotional drama. Drama pulls our vibrations down and that can't be good for us.

Chapter 57: When in a stressful situation…

Your body and your breath are all you have for certain. Think about that for a moment.

- Hold your hands and breathe deeply.
- Try to feel movement in your feet.
- Place your left hand on your heart, right hand on your stomach and breathe deeply.
- Imagine you are in a sphere or bubble. You can see what is going on, but can't be affected by the negative experience of anything outside the bubble.
- Use a Chi ball (Energy ball). Place the palms of the hands facing each other with enough distance to form the sensation of magnetic repulsion. Breathe in and out with the hands facing each other. Deepen the breath and your heart rate will slow down.

- If you are overwhelmed and you are able to get time out, lay flat on the floor in corpse pose. Close your eyes, and bring your attention to your breath.

- **If you have been around a busy/frantic space come out of it, take a deep breath in and out, then draw your arms from the side up to make prayer hands above your head (with inhalation). Hold your breath for as long as you can, then as you exhale out through the mouth, bring the hands down in front of you. Repeat this until you feel better.**

Chapter 58: Take a deep breath

This goes for everything we do.

- **Instead of jumping into an activity, make a point to mark the change from one thing to another.**

- Instead of rushing, take a deep breath and get some form of clarity on why you are rushing/what you are rushing to - do you *have to rush?*

- **Take a deep breath before doing anything different. This is to make sure that you have cleared the energies from the last activity.**

- Take a deep breath before showering, eating, even going to the toilet.

- When we take a deep breath in and out, it shows our mind and body that we are about to begin something slightly different.

- Also, take a deep breath just as you end something too.

- We shallow-breathe too much through the day which increases our heart rate, blood pressure and stress levels. Deep breathing is far more valuable, and does the opposite.

- So, don't forget to consistently take a deep breath.

- You should have done at least 4 or 5 deep breaths whilst reading this chapter.

Chapter 59: Specific exercises targeted to fat loss

All of the exercises we explored above have a positive role. However, ones to include regularly are:

- **HIIT - 7- 10 minutes of High Intensity Interval Training.** I highly recommend **Lucy Wyndham Read** on Youtube. She has a really good library of effective fat loss exercises. Many of her short videos encourage you to do the 7 days a week. I usually just do 6 and have one day off, as my body needs that.

- **Hatha Yoga -** I highly recommend doing Adrienne's 30 day yoga playlists. Again, when I have done this I have one day off a week, as my body feels the need for this. But again, **be your own scientist.**

- **Kundalini Yoga** - For raising your internal energies and it is also an amazing workout. There are kriyas (repetitive breath and movement poses) that are so effective on their own for fat loss. I lost most of my fat with Kundalini yoga; it is intense. Also, look me up on Facebook. I am a qualified Kundalini yoga teacher and I did all my training in India.

- **Yin (Restorative) yoga -** You will need this to balance out all the Yang energy found in other exercise practices! Yin is about stretching the fascia (connective tissue) in a pose for several minutes. It really helps relieve lactic acid and stress in joints and muscles. It is related to physio exercises and there is quite a bit of crossover here, so if you suffer with conditions like sciatica or joint pain, or just can't get on with high intensity exercise, this is for you.

- **Walking -** Walking fast is good for metabolism. It is suggested we should brisk-walk for at least 16 minutes for fat burning. Walking slow is good for mobilising the joints and relaxing. It's good to get some form of walking every day.

Chapter 60: Finally, whatever you decide to do, be true to your inner being.

Whatever you do in life, be true to your inner purpose. Only you can do this.

- The biggest conflict you will ever have is when you are in conflict with yourself.

- Being in conflict with yourself is painful.
- Being in conflict appears like setting good intentions and not feeling the emotional pull to go through with it.
- Your heart wants one thing and your mind wants something else.
- You find it hard to make decisions.
- Your level of anxiety is high.
- **To be true to your inner being, you need to get in touch with what you really want.**
- **How do I know what I really want? When you do something, such as going to the gym, how do you *really* feel?** - I used to be a gym addict until I started developing headaches and intense confusion from how loud and frantic the energies were there. When I took up yoga instead, I felt more space develop in my head, so I knew that the gym is just not for me. We are all different, so don't cancel your membership just because you've read this book! But you need to know if you really do belong there. If you go there because your friends do but you always come away feeling unsatisfied, then leave. It needs to resonate with *you*.
- **You may even experience the same thing about a job you thought you enjoyed.** You might find after a while that your inner being lets you know you are not meant for your job by giving you clammy hands before leaving the house. You may experience a sense of dread. You may also experience stomach discomforts or even bowel problems. Don't just treat these as isolated things to go to the doctor for. If

there is a cause, then address the cause, not the symptom, and the symptom should go pretty quickly. Of course if it doesn't, then see what your doc has to say… but remember, **approach all this intelligently, as someone in charge of your own body and mind.** You know your own body better than any doctor does. If you eat badly, exercise too much or not enough or in the wrong way, live with the wrong people or have the wrong job, then chances are you are making your own health problems. **<u>Stress is the number one cause of 'Western' diseases like heart disease, diabetes, cancer.</u> Cut the stress, clean up your act and things will improve.** Stress pills just prolong the problem and make it more likely you will end up very, very ill one day.

- **This is why, in what ever you do, pay attention to what your body tells you about any situation. This can prevent stress, which we know prevents those stress hormones from rising and all that follows.**

Final words – A Rule of thumb

- Be inquisitive in your life - whether it's for fat loss or anything else.
- Make health your priority - fat loss will be a welcome side effect of better health.
- Cut out processed and junk food.
- Cut out white/refined sugar and flour.
- Add more greens (200g with every meal).
- Eat more healthy protein.
- Quit <u>all</u> sodas/soft drinks - they do you no good. That goes for energy drinks too. You only need water, and what nature has already given us.
- Drink lots more water!
- Avoid pollutants and BPA bottles - due to hormonal influences.
- **Go plant based** - animal proteins cause fat retention and are full of hormones and antibiotics. At the very

least, cut all red meats and go over to white meats. In time, see where you can go from there.

- **Move more** - and I don't mean going to the gym.
- **Find ways to live stress free.**
- **Listen to your gut.**
- **Clear your mind daily.**
- **Everything is trial and error - find a way that suits you.**
- **If you indulge, enjoy it, thrive on it - but understand the consequences and cut back right away the next day.**
- **Don't dwell on negativity.**
- **Do what makes you happy** as long as you know it is also right.
- **Enjoy life!**

Reference list

- The Science of Skinny - Dee McCaffrey
- Freedom from the diet trap - Jason Vale
- Reboot Juice diet - Joe Cross
- Gamechanger - Netflix
- Cowspiracy - Netflix
- Seaspiracy - Netflix

- A Plastic Ocean - Netflix
- What the Health - Netflix
- Michael Mosley on the 5:2 Fasting diet (You may want to do some researching on Google and Youtube). There are articles and websites, the initial program doesn't appear to be there on Youtube.
- Fat, Sick and Nearly Dead by Joe Cross - Netflix/Youtube
- Superjuice Me by Jason Vale - Youtube
- Lose weight Now - Dr. Jade Teta
- Inner Engineering - Sadhguru
- 112 Meditations for self-realisation - Ranjit Chaudhri
- Kundalini Tantra - Swami Satyananda Saraswati

If you would like help in your fat loss journey, please get in touch with me via email: **kundaliniwithkatrina@gmail.com**

Printed in Great Britain
by Amazon